HOLIDAY MANDALAS

CHRISTMAS MANDALAS

AN ADVENT CALENDAR

This book belongs to:

Beate Kumar

Bibi LeBlanc

Culture to Color Holiday Wellness Series

Printed in the USA

First Edition

Cover Design & Interior by
Culture to Color, LLC

ISBN: 978-1-7337985-8-7

To order in bulk contact publisher,
CultureToColor.com

For more information visit:
CultureToColor.com

CS@CultureToColor.com
386-228-5147

CHRISTMAS MANDALAS

WELCOME TO BOOK 1 IN THE CULTURE TO COLOR HOLIDAY WELLNESS SERIES.

MANDALAS

The word *mandala* is derived from Sanskrit and means circle.
The typically circular designs represent the universe
and symbolize the idea that life is never-ending
and everything is connected.

CHRISTMAS IS A SPECIAL TIME OF THE YEAR!

We hear a lot about the spirit of Christmas, we feel it, we look forward
to it. And though it means slightly different things to each of us,
there seem to be common threads weaving through our stories
and family traditions. Christmas is a time for togetherness,
reflection and acceptance, and the desire
to spread love and happiness, peace and joy.

*May your Christmas sparkle with love,
laughter, and goodwill. And may the year ahead
be full of contentment and joy.*

Bibi & Beate

*P.S. We would love to see your colored images.
Please send them to us at bibi@culturetocolor.com
or post them on social media
with hashtags #culturetocolor*

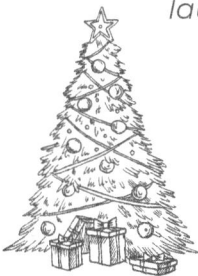

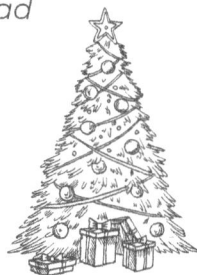

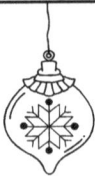

WELLNESS BENEFITS OF COLORING

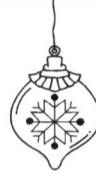

If you include coloring in your daily routine, you will find
it has many benefits for *you*, the coloring artist.
To name just a few, coloring:

IMPROVES FOCUS

Coloring requires repetition and attention to detail. It opens up
your brain's frontal lobe, which controls organizing
and problem-solving, and allows you to focus on the activity
rather than your worries.

REDUCES STRESS AND ANXIETY

Coloring relaxes the fear center (amygdala) in your brain,
putting you in a state similar to meditation. Coloring mandalas
helps remove irritating thoughts and allows the creative mind
to run free and relax.

IMPROVES SLEEP

Coloring as your bedtime ritual instead of using electronics can
lead to a better night's sleep. The light emitted by electronic
devices lowers the level of Melatonin, your sleep hormone,
whereas coloring does not affect your Melatonin level.

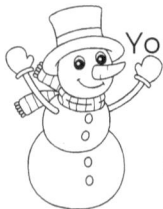

You can take coloring supplies anywhere. And you don't
have to be an artist or an expert to color and
create something beautiful. Seeing your finished
coloring page provides a sense of accomplishment.

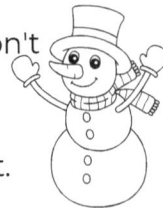

I

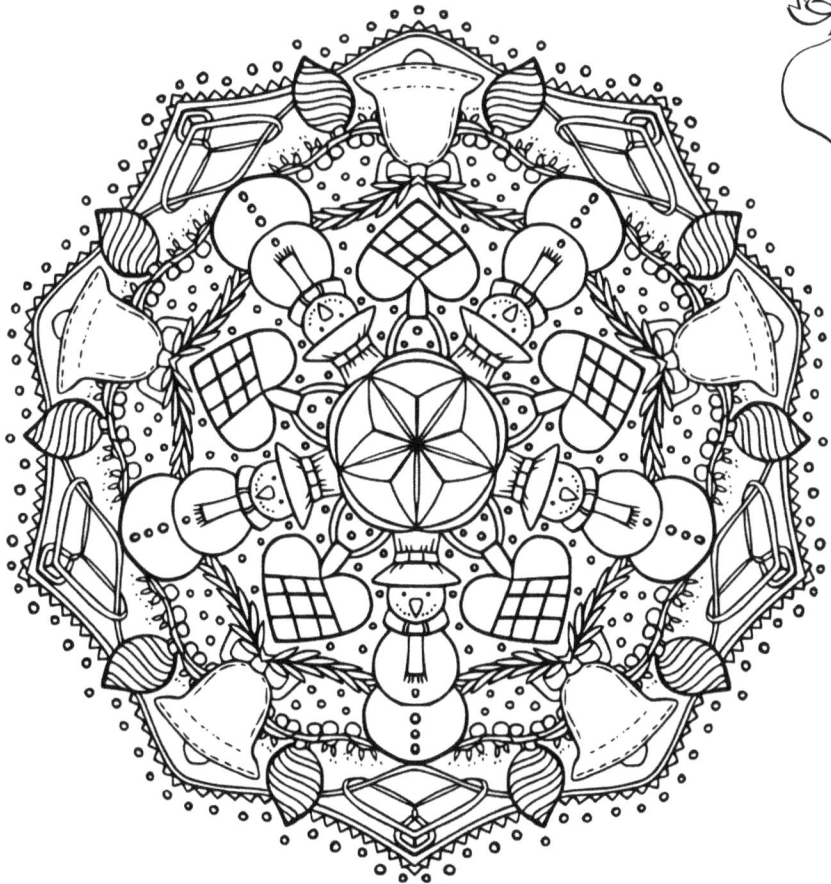

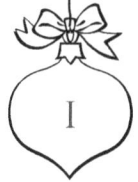

"IT'S THE MOST WONDERFUL TIME OF THE YEAR."
EDWARD POLA & GEORGE WYLE

2

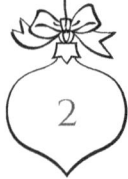

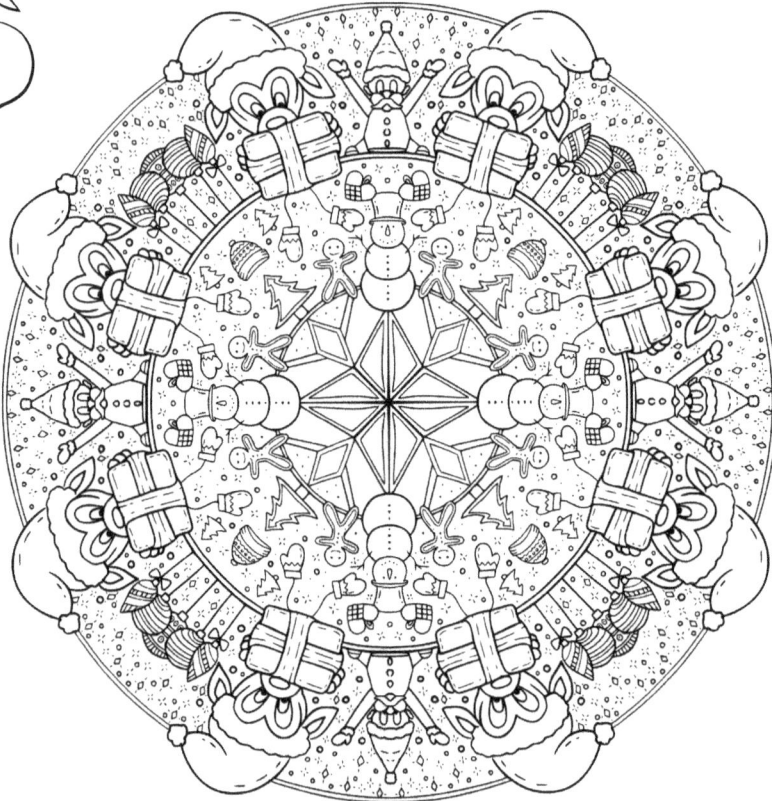

"CHRISTMAS IS MOST TRULY CHRISTMAS WHEN WE CELEBRATE IT
BY GIVING THE LIGHT OF LOVE TO THOSE WHO NEED IT MOST."
RUTH CARTER STAPLETON

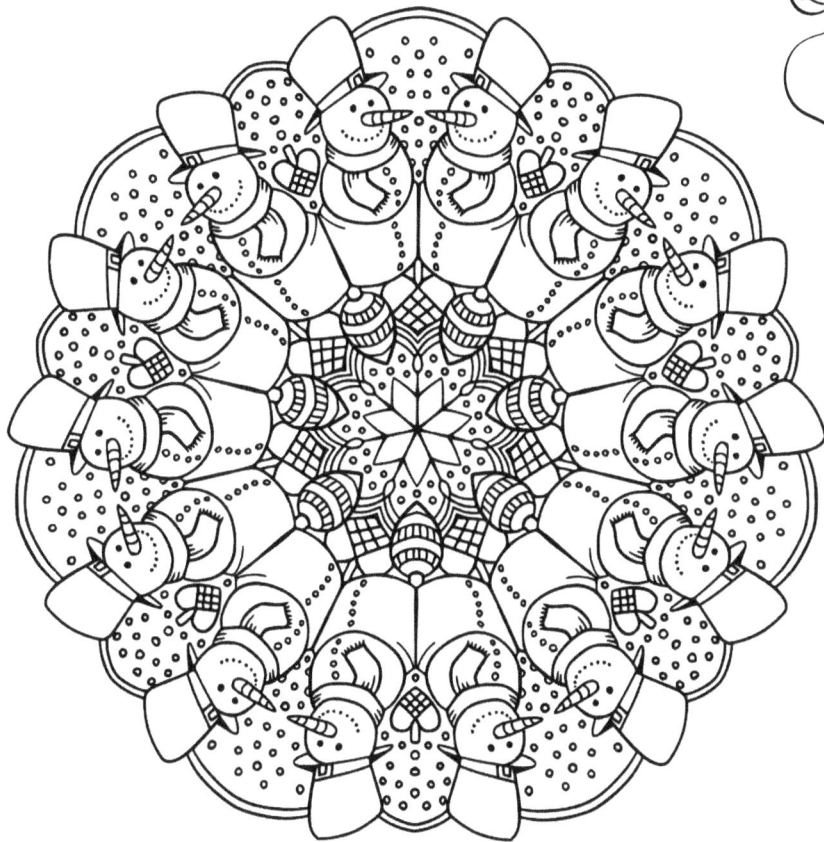

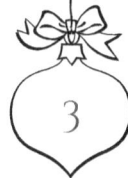

"A JOY THAT IS SHARED IS A JOY MADE DOUBLE."
JOHN ROY

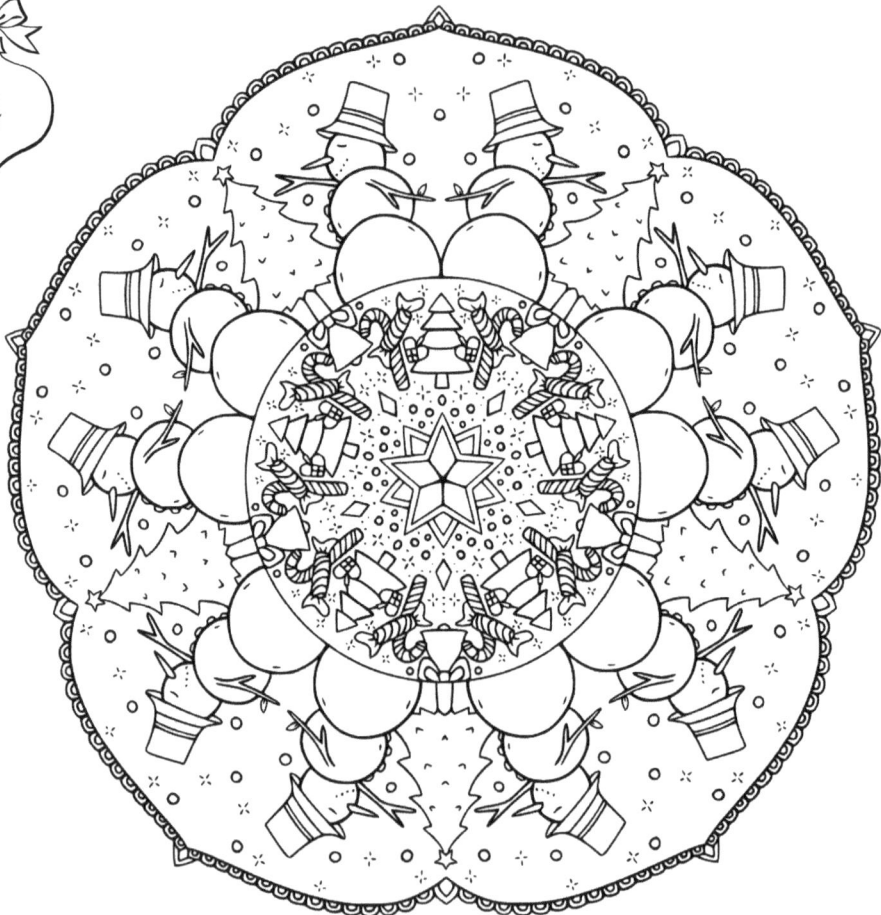

4

"SNOW IS THE CHRISTMAS SEASON'S FAIRY DUST."

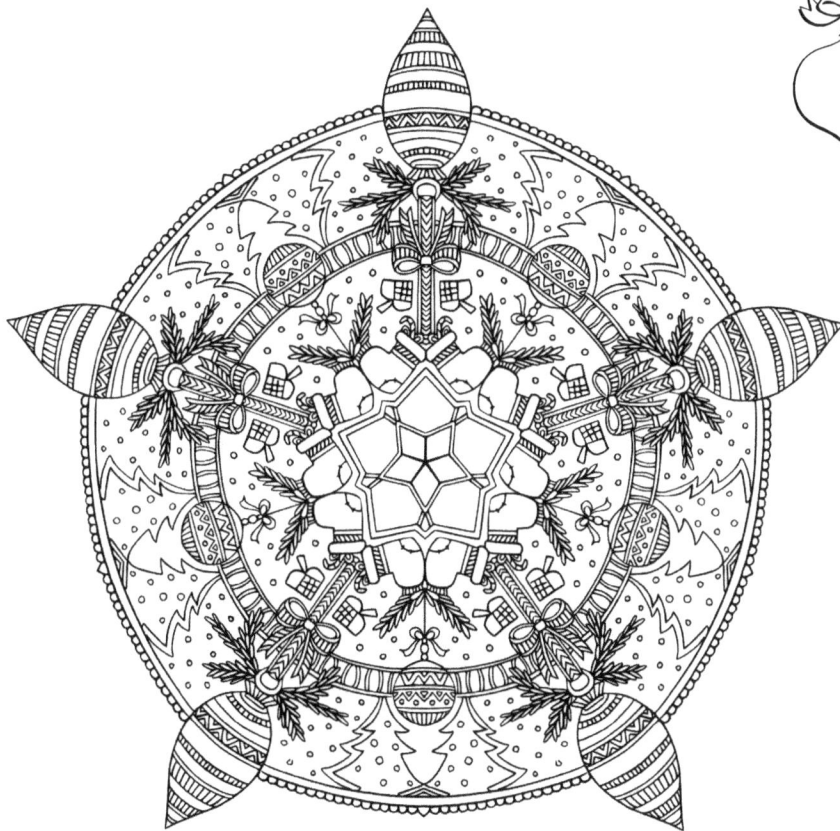

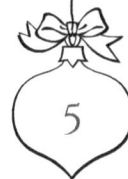

"CHRISTMAS IS A SEASON NOT ONLY OF REJOICING,
BUT OF REFLECTION."
WINSTON CHURCHILL

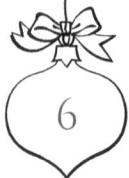

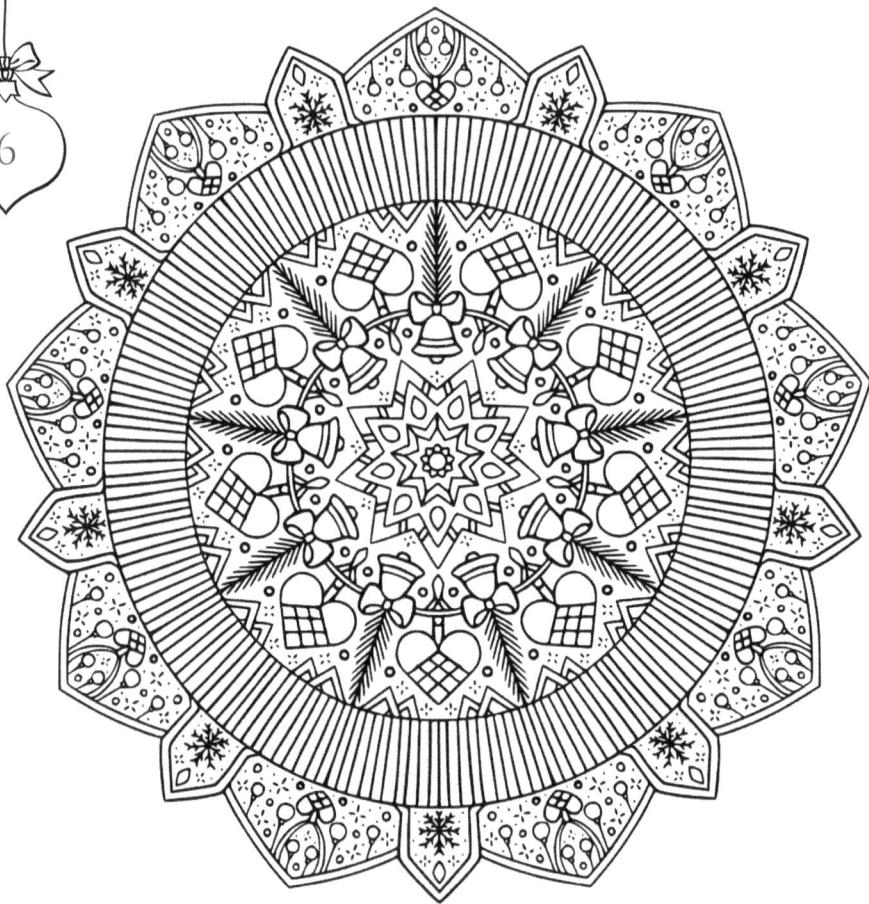

"CHRISTMAS WILL ALWAYS BE AS LONG AS THE CHRISTMAS SPIRIT
IS A SPIRIT OF GIVING AND FORGIVING."
J. C. PENNEY

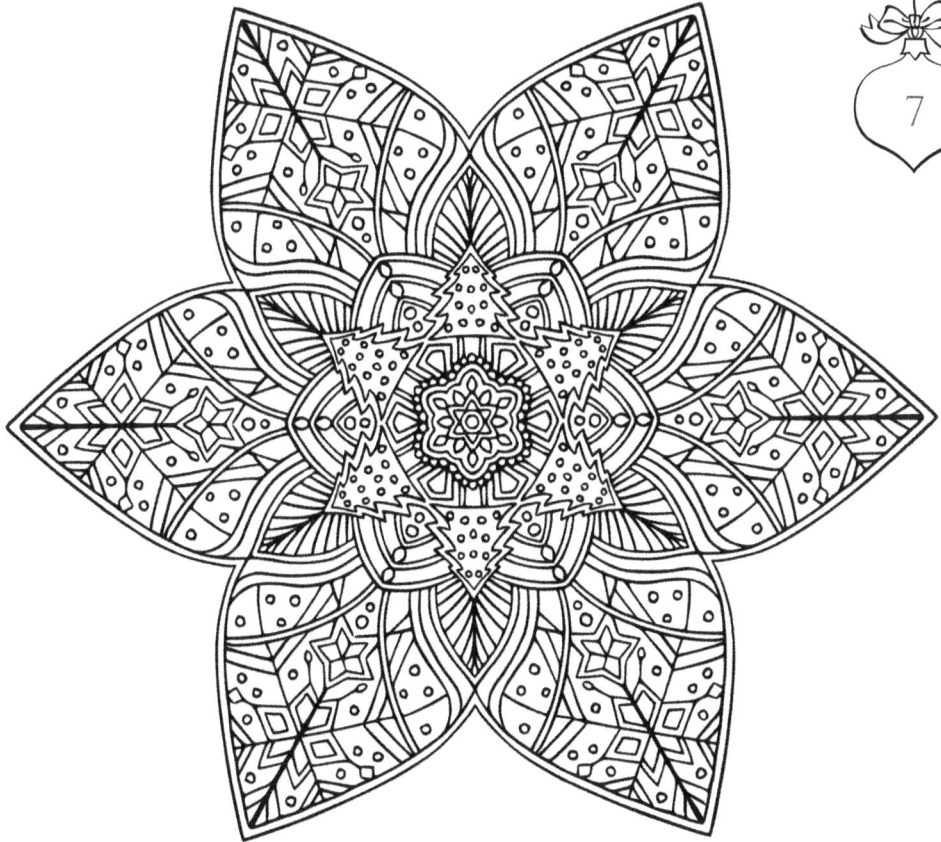

"I WILL HONOR CHRISTMAS IN MY HEART,
AND TRY TO KEEP IT ALL THE YEAR."
CHARLES DICKENS

8

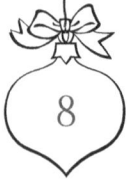

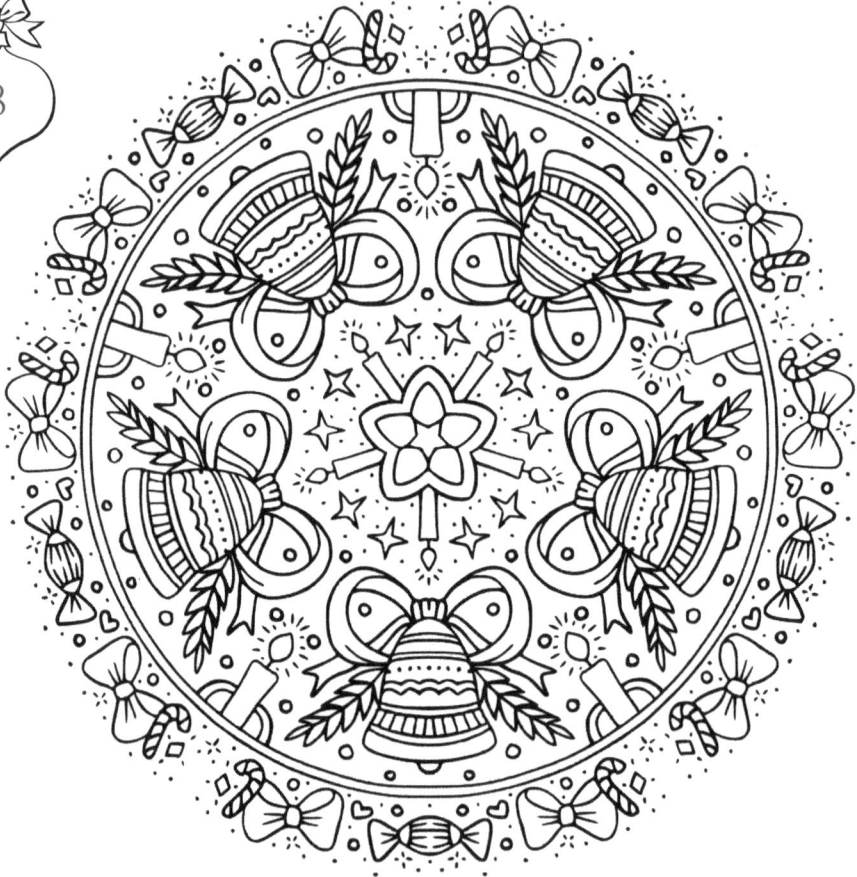

"EVERY TIME A BELL RINGS AN ANGEL GETS HIS WINGS."
IT'S A WONDERFUL LIFE

9

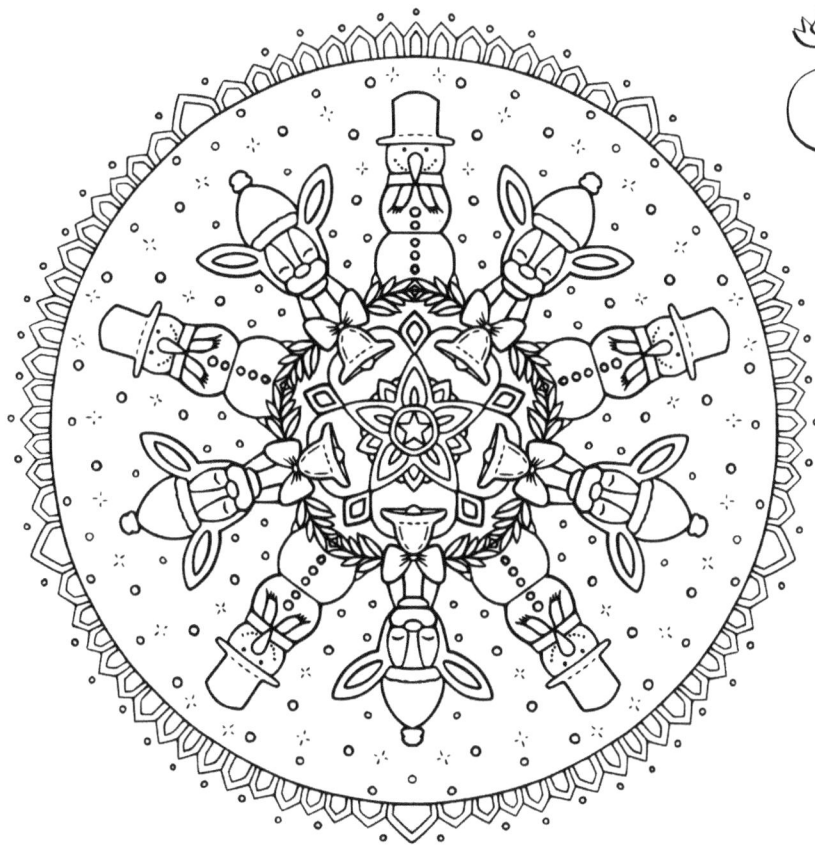

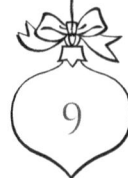

"GIFTS OF TIME AND LOVE ARE SURELY
THE BASIC INGREDIENTS OF A TRULY MERRY CHRISTMAS."
PEG BRACKEN

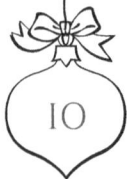

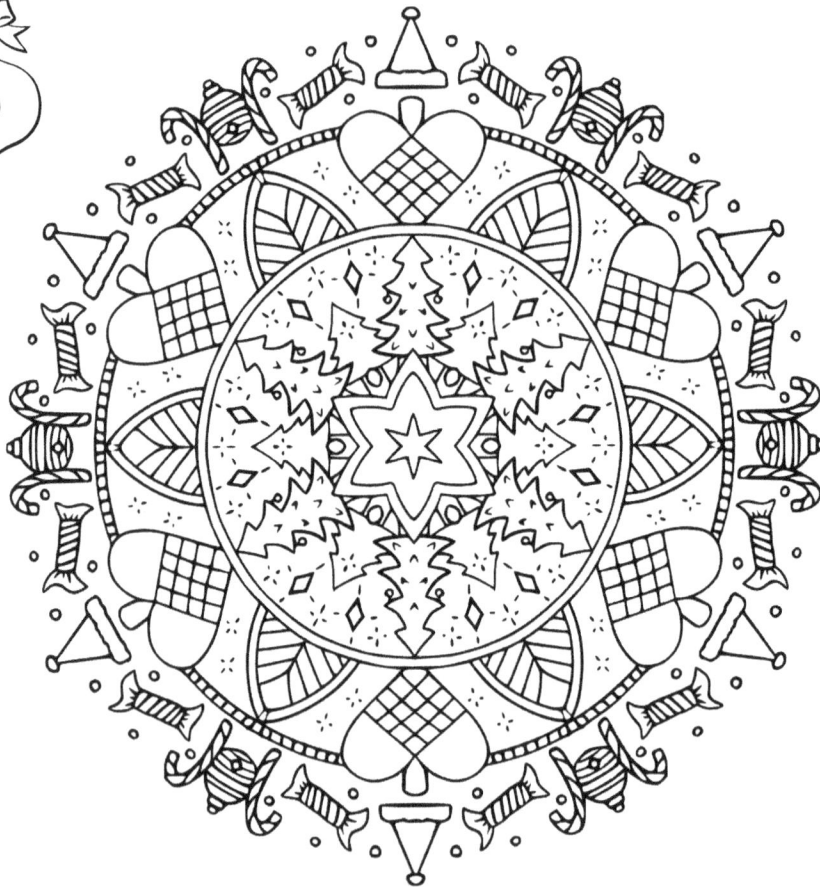

"IT IS CHRISTMAS IN THE HEART
THAT PUTS CHRISTMAS IN THE AIR."
W.T. ELLIS

II

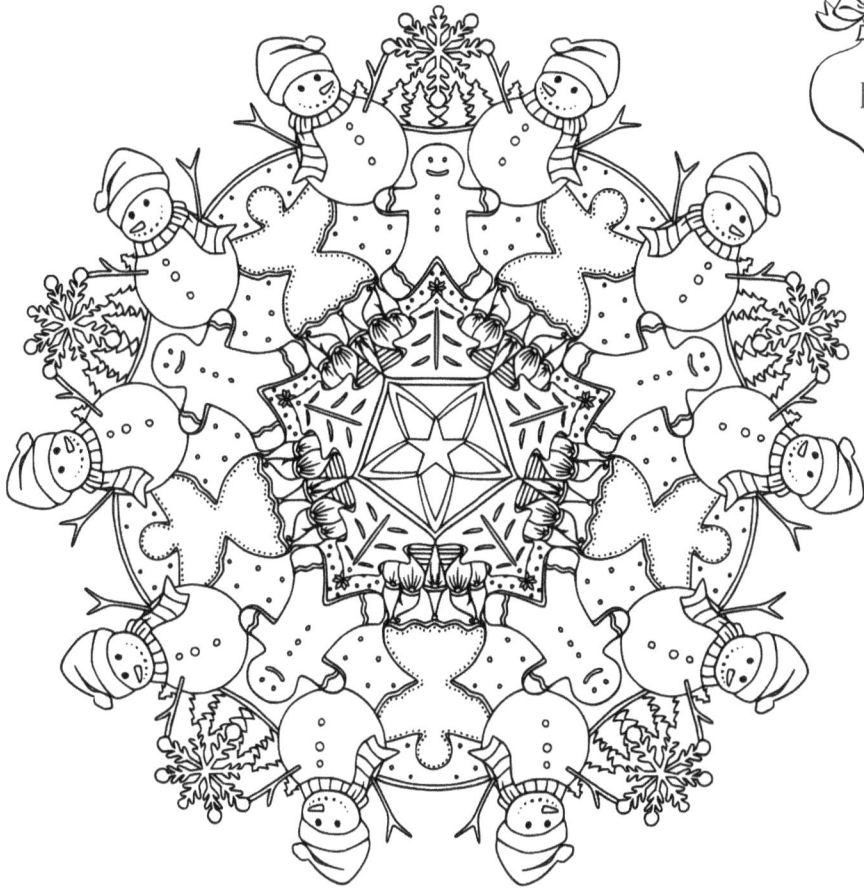

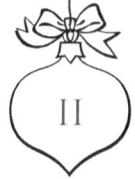

"'TIS THE SEASON TO BE JOLLY!"
DECK THE HALLS

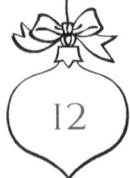

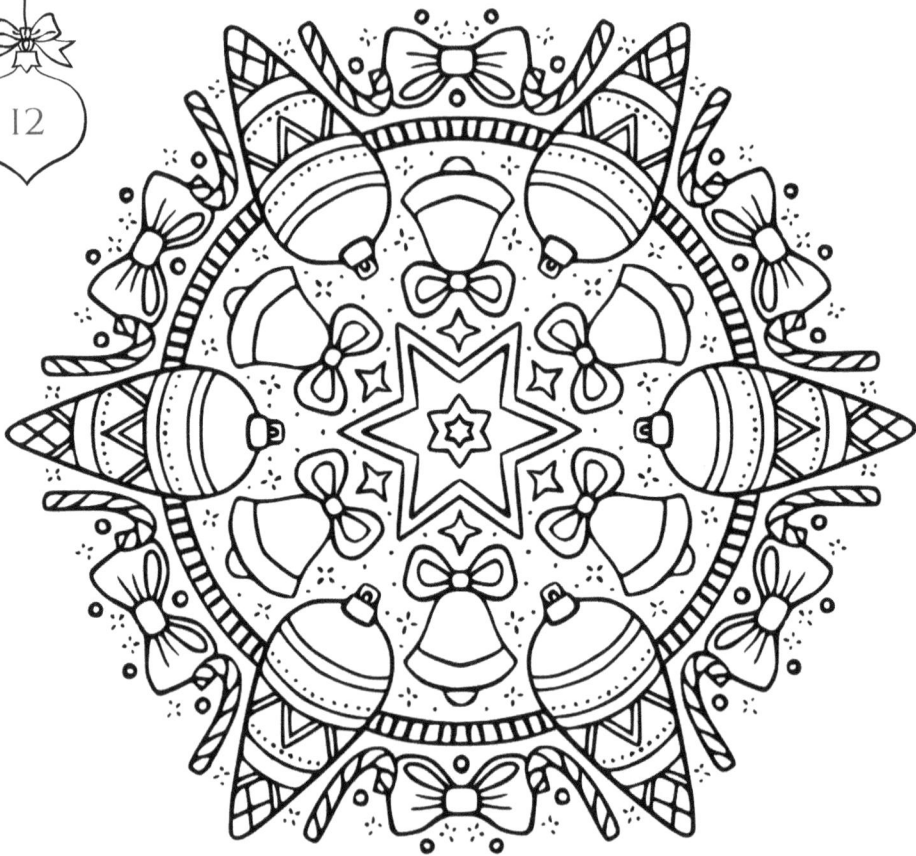

"MAY YOUR DAYS BE MERRY AND BRIGHT."
WHITE CHRISTMAS

13

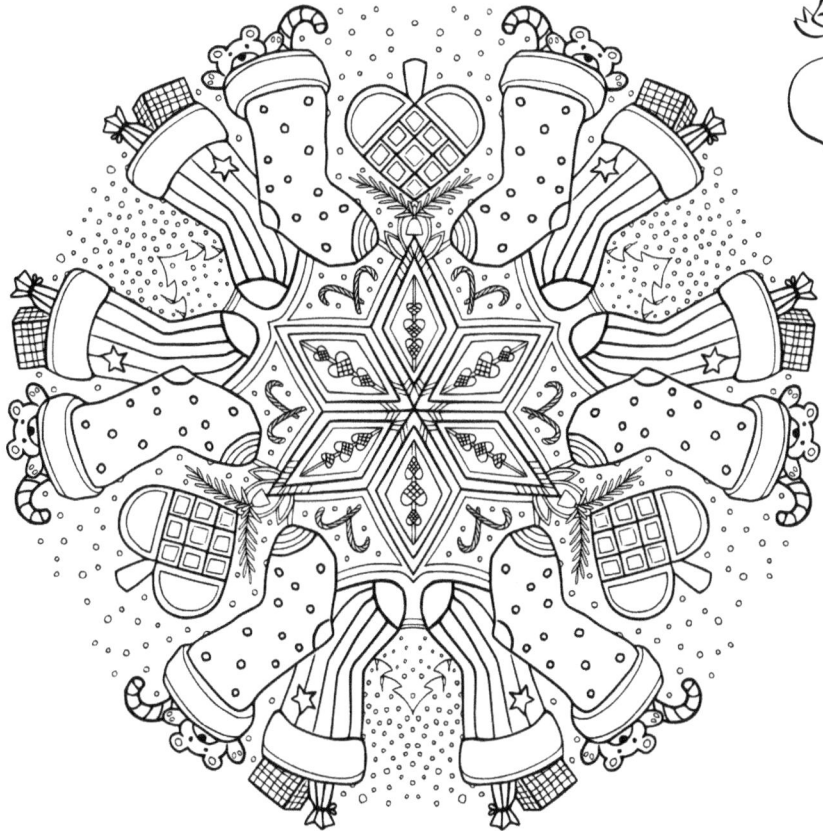

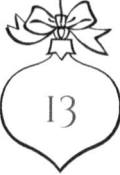

"CHRISTMAS, MY CHILD, IS LOVE IN ACTION.
EVERY TIME WE LOVE, EVERY TIME WE GIVE, IT'S CHRISTMAS."
DALE EVANS ROGERS

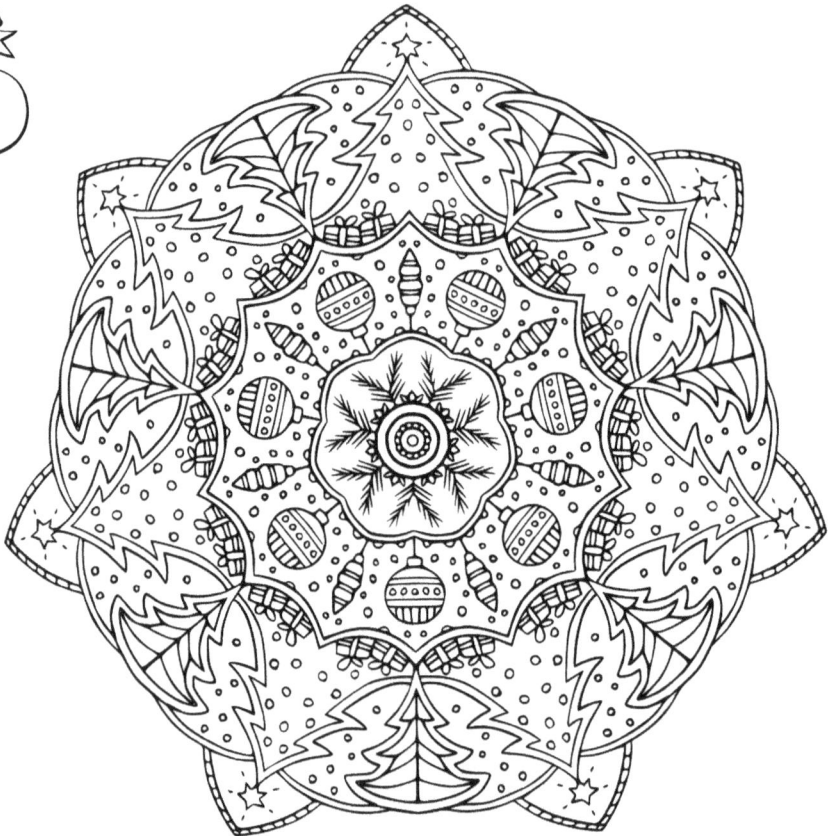

14

"MAY THE SPIRIT OF CHRISTMAS BRING YOU PEACE,
THE GLADNESS OF CHRISTMAS GIVE YOU HOPE,
THE WARMTH OF CHRISTMAS GRANT YOU LOVE."
UNKNOWN

15

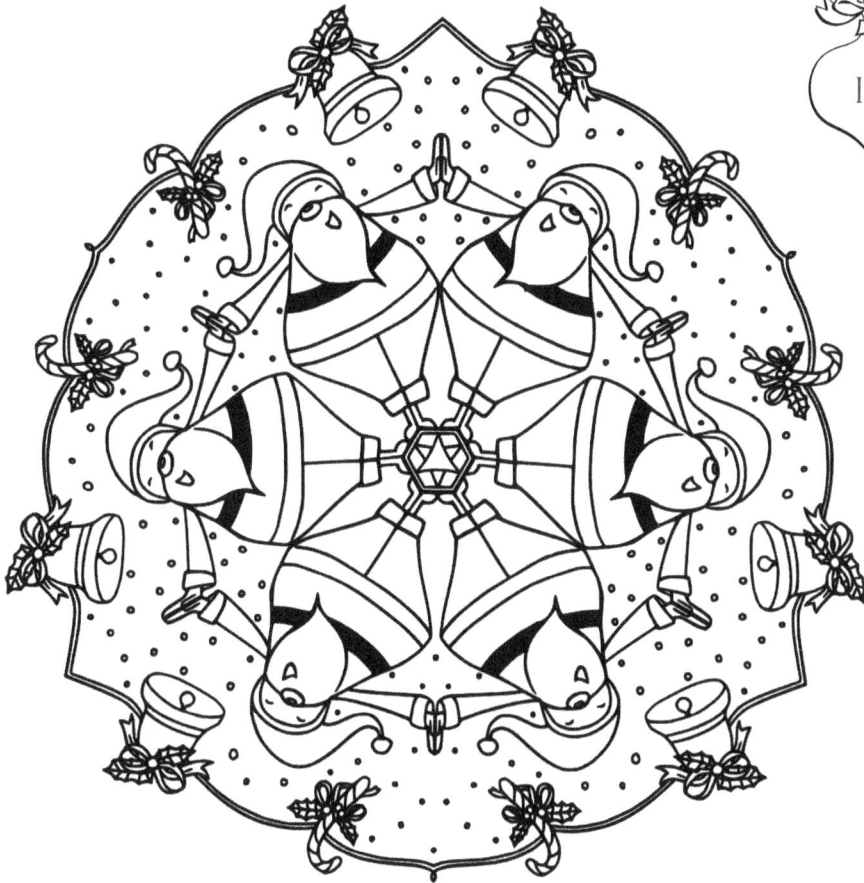

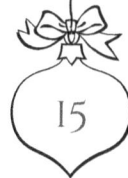

"CHRISTMAS IS A TOGETHER-Y SORT OF HOLIDAY."
WINNIE THE POOH

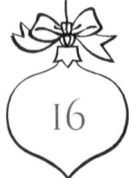

16

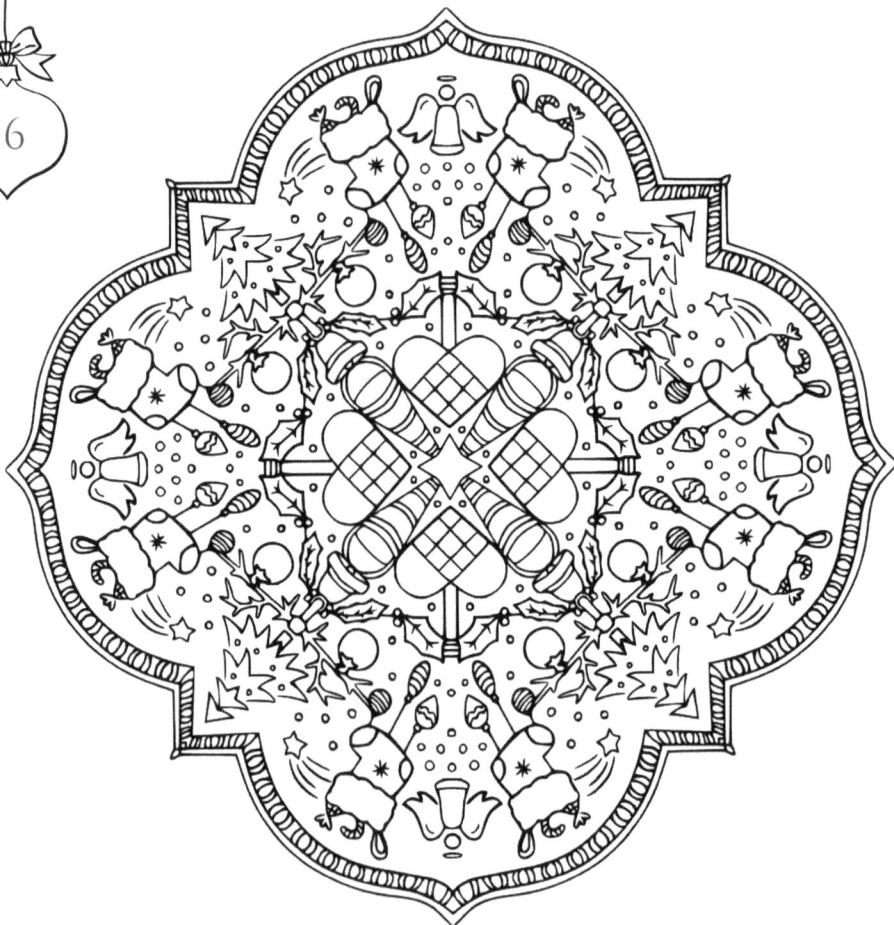

"THE JOY OF BRIGHTENING OTHER LIVES BECOMES FOR US THE
MAGIC OF THE HOLIDAYS."
W.C. JONES

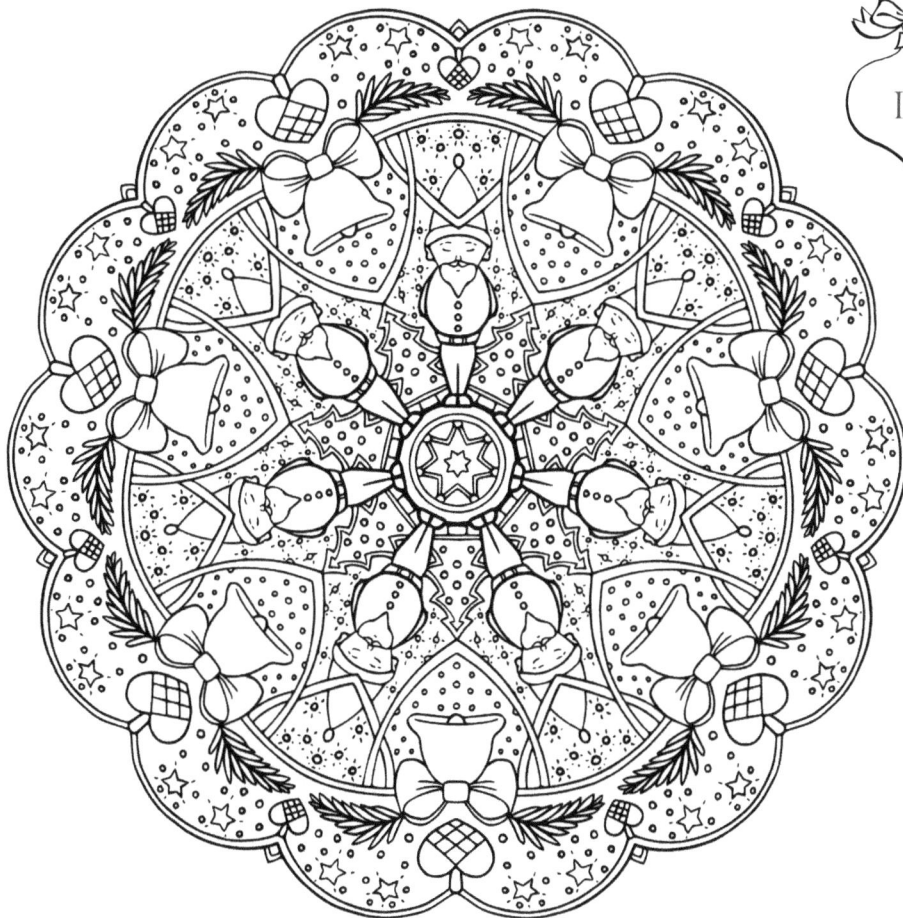

17

"CHRISTMAS WAVES A MAGIC WAND OVER THIS WORLD,
AND BEHOLD, EVERYTHING IS SOFTER AND MORE BEAUTIFUL."
NORMAN VINCENT PEALE

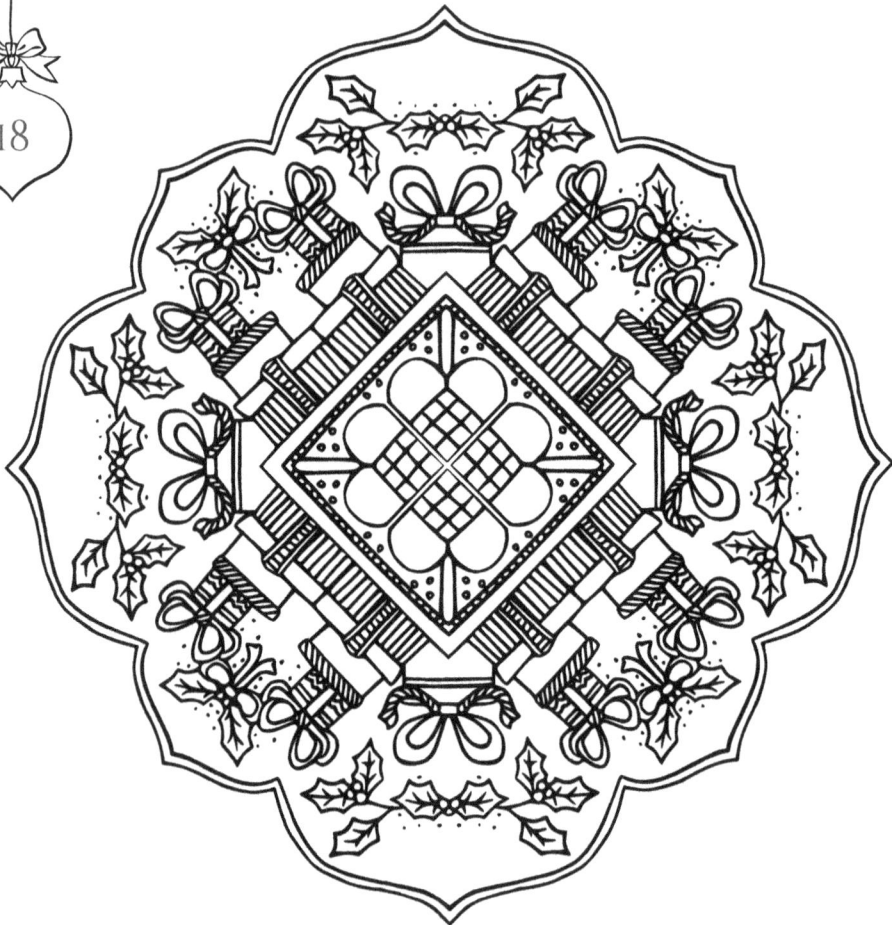

18

"CHRISTMAS IS NOT AS MUCH ABOUT OPENING OUR PRESENTS
AS OPENING OUR HEARTS."
JANICE MAEDITERE

19

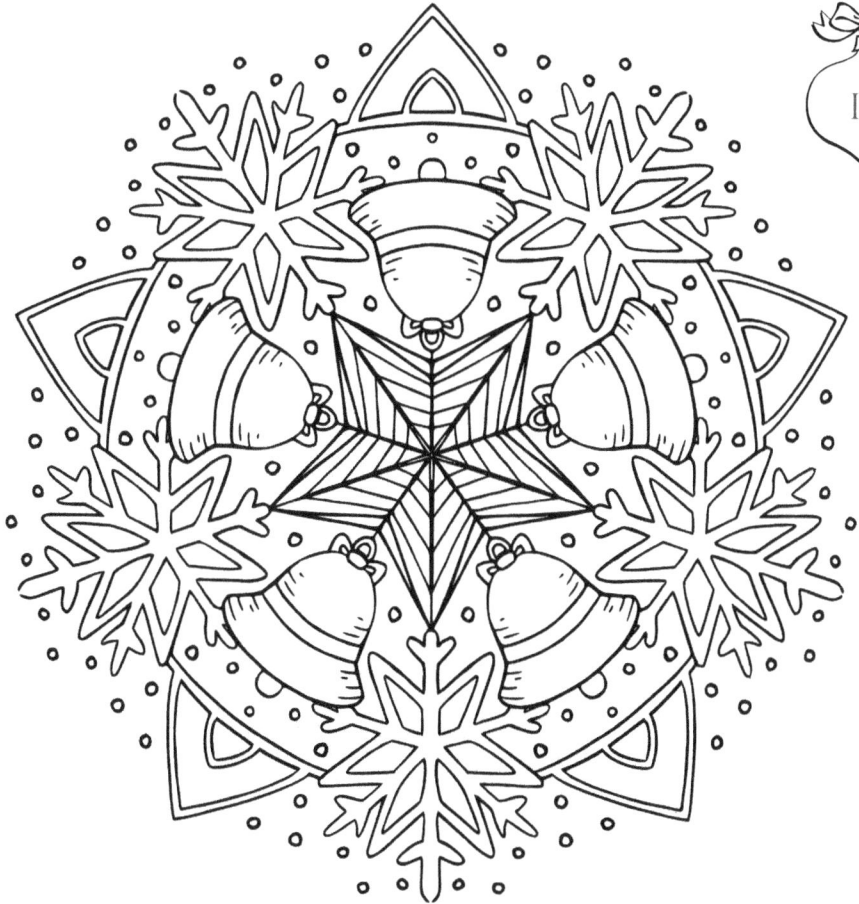

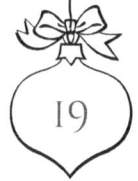

"I HEARD THE BELLS ON CHRISTMAS DAY
THEIR OLD, FAMILIAR CAROLS PLAY."
HENRY WADSWORTH LONGFELLOW

20

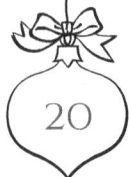

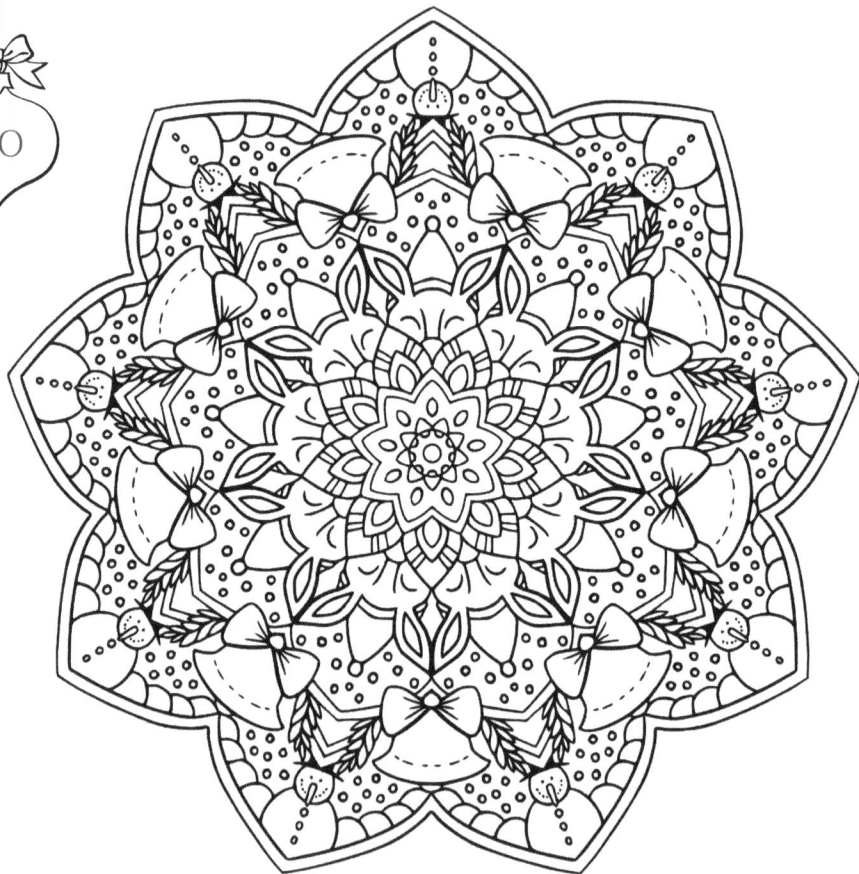

"THE WARMTH AND JOY OF CHRISTMAS
BRING US CLOSER TO EACH OTHER."
EMILY MATTHEWS

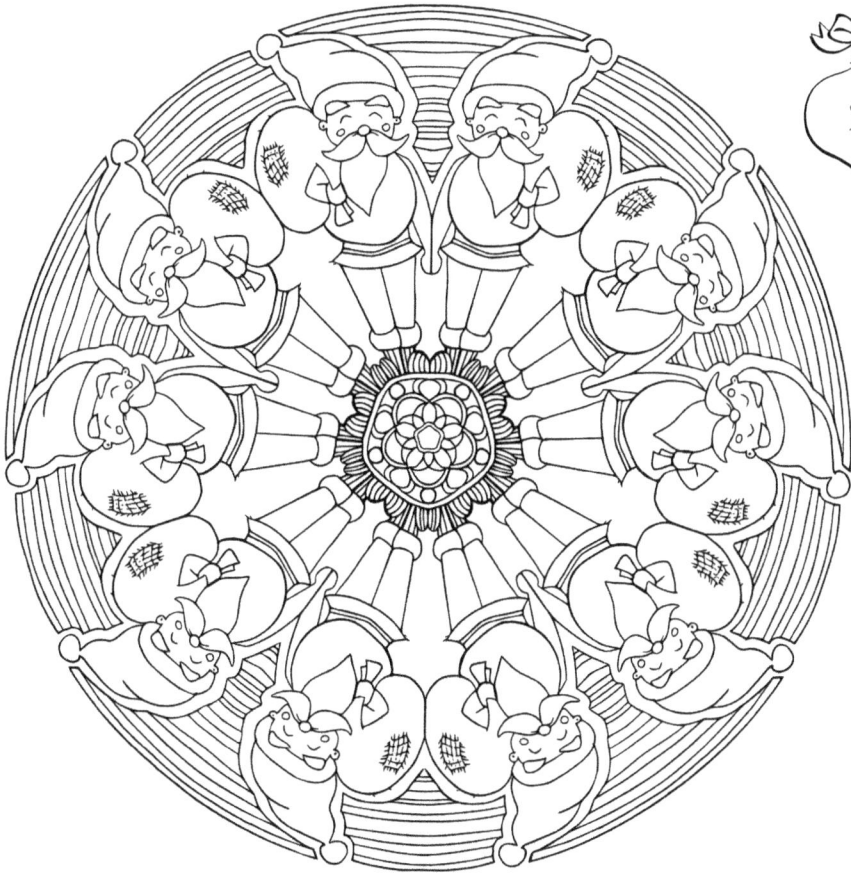

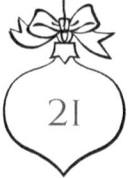

21

"CHRISTMAS WILL ALWAYS BE AS LONG
AS WE STAND HEART TO HEART AND HAND IN HAND."
DR. SEUSS

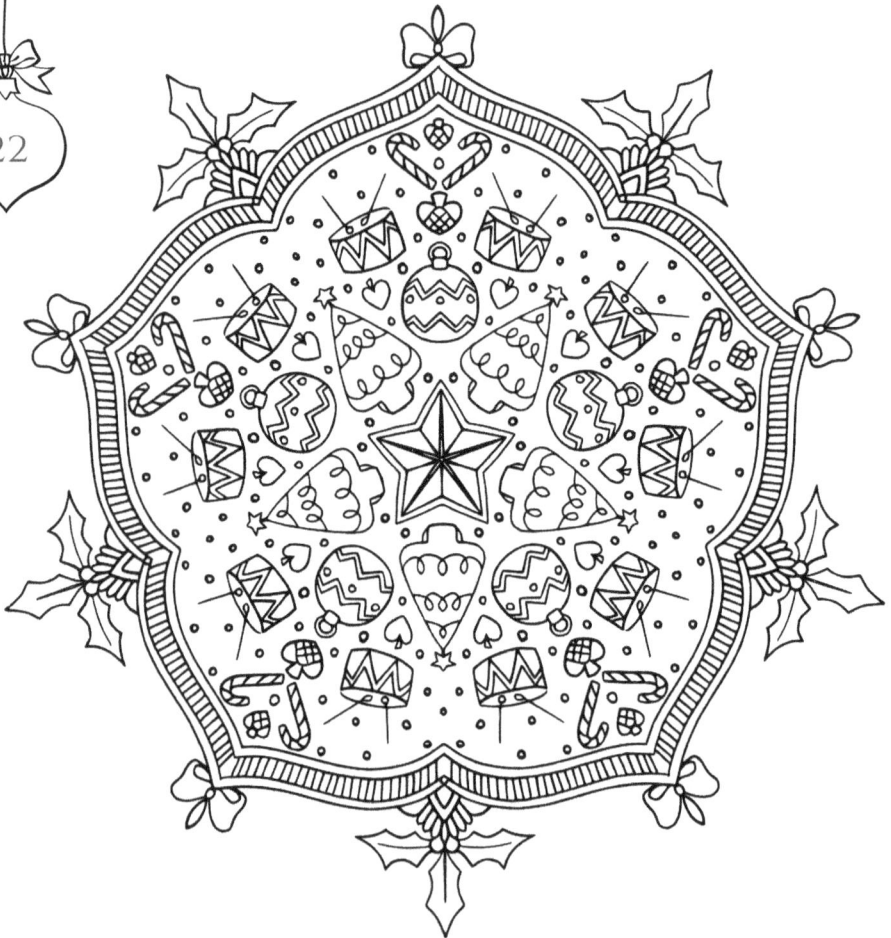

22

"AT CHRISTMAS, ALL ROADS LEAD HOME."
MARJORIE HOLMES

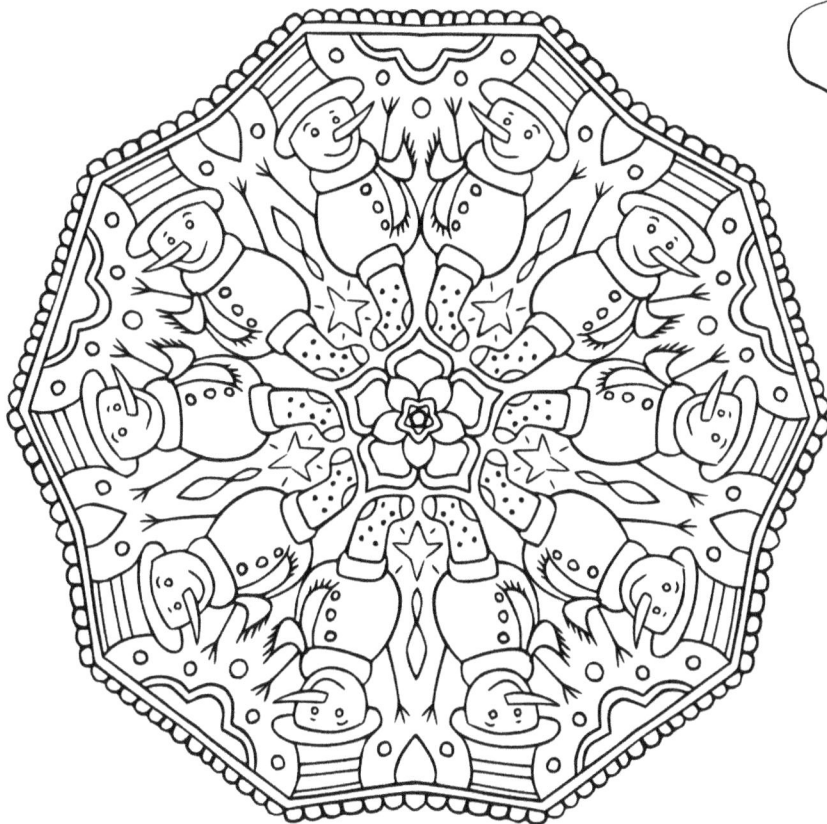

23

"I'M DREAMING OF A WHITE CHRISTMAS."
IRVING BERLIN

24

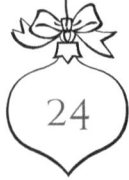

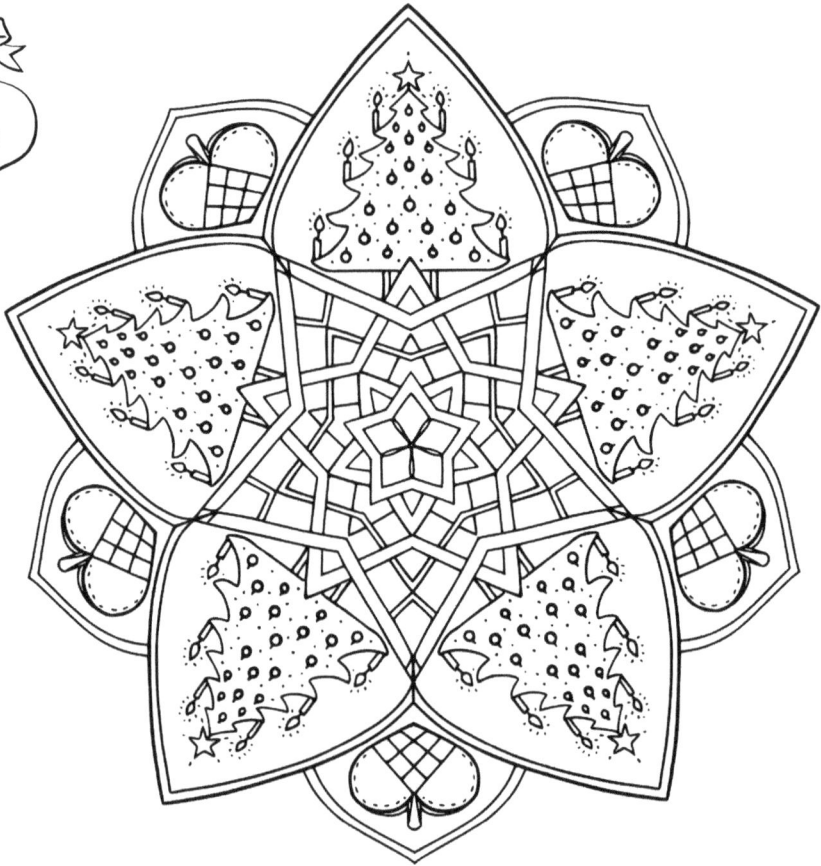

MAY YOUR CHRISTMAS SPARKLE WITH MOMENTS OF LOVE, LAUGHTER AND
GOODWILL. AND MAY THE YEAR AHEAD BE FULL OF CONTENTMENT AND JOY.
MERRY CHRISTMAS!

Bibi & Beate

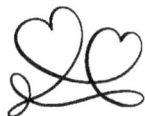

OUR STORY

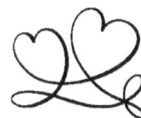

My sister Beate and I grew up together
in West Berlin, Germany.

Our life paths led us in opposite directions;
she married and moved to India, I married and moved to the U.S.

Even though we live far apart, we are very close
and usually meet once a year in Berlin.

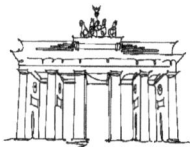

One of Beate's greatest joys is coloring mandalas,
and we started creating cards and books in sister-Zoom sessions.
This labor of love brings us even closer together.

We hope you enjoyed this book!

Love from our ♡ homes to yours!

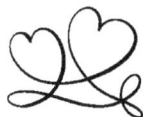

Bibi

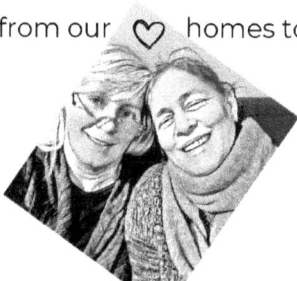

Beate

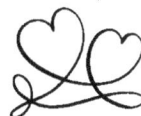

This book was created by best-selling author and winner of the
FAPA President's Book Award &
finalist in the *Eric Hoffer International Book Award*
for her book
Explore the Sights of Berlin Divided - Berlin United

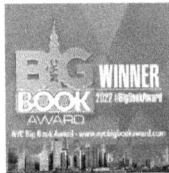

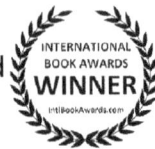

∂

Kops-Fetherling International Book Award for
Discover Food & Wine of Tuscany, Italy

∂

Purple Dragonfly International Book Award &
International Book Award &
IBPA Benjamin Franklin Book Award &
FAPA President's Book Award for
Endangered Animals of North America/
Bedrohte Tiere Nordamerikas

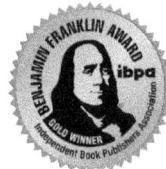

∂

Next Generation International Indie Book Award &
Purple Dragonfly International Book Award &
FAPA President's Book Award for
Explore the Sights of San Francisco, Chinatown

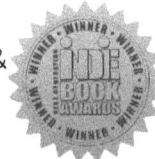

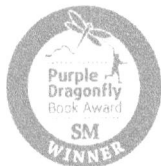

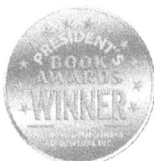

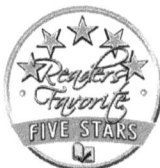

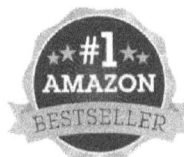

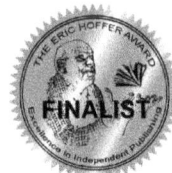

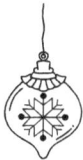

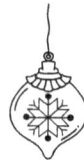

PLEASE VISIT
ETSY.COM/SHOP/CULTURETOCOLOR

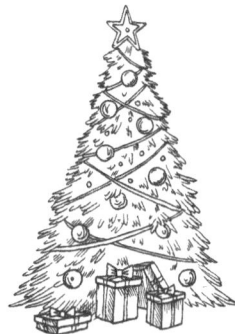

FOR COLORING INSPIRATION
AND MANDALA CARDS

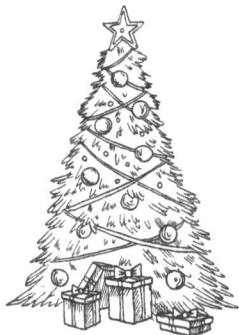

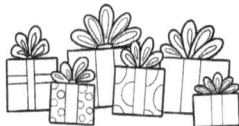

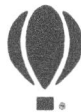

Culture to Color

#ConnectingCulturesThroughColoring!

ABOUT CULTURE TO COLOR

For more information visit CultureToColor.com

Tag us with your colored pages #CultureToColor

Follow us on:

(f) facebook.com/CultureToColor

(⊙) instagram.com/Culture_To_Color

(in) linkedin.com/in/bibileblanc

Contact us

Bibi LeBlanc

cs@culturetocolor.com

386-309-2632

TITLES AVAILABLE IN THE CULTURE TO COLOR BOOK SERIES

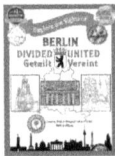

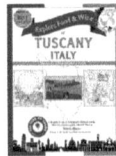

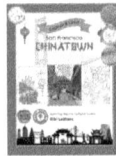

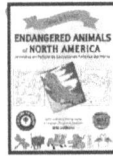

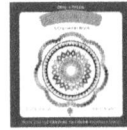

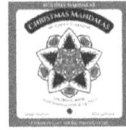

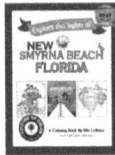

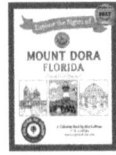

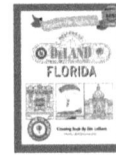

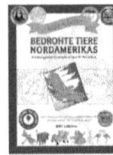

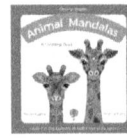

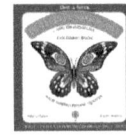

www.ingramcontent.com/pod-product-compliance
Lightning Source LLC
Chambersburg PA
CBHW042250040426

42337CB00046B/5188